We're thrilled you're reading this book.

Congratulations – if you're reading this, you've taken the first step toward better overall health and living the life you want.

In this book, the doctors of ClearChoice will share with you 27 "insider" tips to help you achieve a healthy smile that will last a lifetime. It's our gift to you!

Enjoy our little book about huge smiles. Soon, your smile will be bigger and brighter than ever.

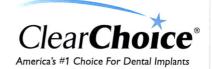

It's from your ClearChoice doctors—acknowledged leaders in the field of dental implants.

In fact, we're America's #1 choice for dental implants.

It's all we do.

But this book is not about ClearChoice.

It's about the things you need to know about the biggest breakthrough in dentistry in the past twenty-five years: dental implants.

Most people don't know anything about them.

Which means that millions of people are living with constant, unnecessary pain and discomfort.

Not to mention all the embarrassment and limitations that come with bad teeth.

Or, worse yet, dentures.

What you'll find here is a lot of useful information about sensible new procedures that are dramatically changing people's lives for the better.

Procedures that can replace a single tooth or a whole mouthful with implants that look and feel like natural teeth.

We hope you'll enjoy reading this.

You're one step closer to the magic moment when you wake up and look in the mirror at the beautiful smile you deserve.

— **The ClearChoice Alliance of Oral Surgeons and Prosthodontists**

Lesson 1

Give your mouth a hand.

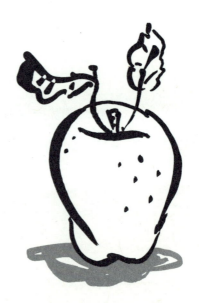

If you're missing a tooth or teeth, it's embarrassing.

It hurts. It hurts your self-confidence. Your relationships. And your work.

It makes life painful.

There are days when just looking at apples, carrots, and steak makes you want to cry.

Well, here are two things you need to know:

<u>First</u>, you are not alone.

By the age of 50, many people will lose four or more teeth.

Which means you are among the millions of Americans suffering from missing, loose, or painful teeth, and weak or troublesome gums.

And, if you do nothing, it usually will only get worse.

<u>Second</u>, there is now something you can do about it.

There's a quiet dental revolution going on.

Permanent replacement teeth are available—and affordable because of breakthroughs in materials and procedures.

What was once an option for only the very wealthy is now available to millions of Americans— along with the deep emotional satisfaction and self-esteem that come from eating, talking, and smiling with a confidence you haven't felt in years.

Welcome to your new smile.

Lesson 2

The blame game: your parents.

Perhaps you should blame your folks.

Much of our dental health is inherited, and no amount of brushing, flossing, or trips to the dentist can outsmart your genetics.

It turns out that a lot of people with dental problems are actually sticklers about their oral health.

So, if your teeth are prone to decay or are too crooked, or if you've got gum disease, these could be unwelcome gifts from your ancestors.

It's also possible you inherited soft enamel, which probably means your teeth are deteriorating or are filled or crowned.

Don't be too angry, because you don't have to suffer.

Unlike your parents' generation, you can do something to permanently correct many of the dental gifts they did—or didn't—provide.

Now you have the option to do something positive to relieve your "hereditary burden."

Lesson 3

The blame game: your age.

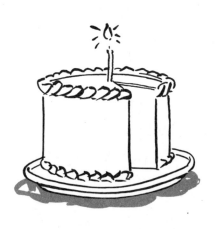

People are living longer lives than ever. The trouble is, many of us are simply outliving our teeth.

As we age, our teeth become worn, stained, and brittle. They lose luster, get yellow, and are susceptible to cracks and breaks. Over time, they wear from daily chewing and from what we eat and drink.

It's worse if we grind our teeth and clench our jaws.

In addition to our teeth, as gums age, they recede and expose the roots of the teeth, so that they aren't protected.

The effects of all these things on our teeth are cumulative—they add up little by little, year by year.

This leads to a decline in the fiber content and blood vessels of the gums, so teeth loosen, gums bleed, and things break and fall out.

Consider it the price you pay for longevity.

It's well worth it, and now you can do something about the dental downside of living a long life.

Lesson 4

The blame game: your competitors.

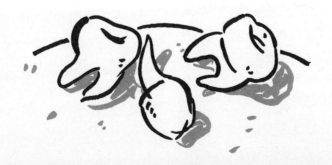

Baseball. Soccer. Hockey. Trampolines. Dirt bikes.

It's astonishing the ways people find to lose teeth.

Sometimes it's competitors.

Sometimes we do it to ourselves, thank you.

The problem is this: Teeth depend on other teeth.

It's a buddy system.

They draw strength from one another, support each other, and keep our jawbones healthy. When one or more fall out, the teeth around it are weakened. It even weakens the bone above or below. Without teeth or roots there to stimulate the growth of bone, our bones start to disappear.

Worse, this deterioration weakens adjacent teeth, resulting in a domino effect.

In sum, one lost tooth often means more will eventually follow.

(Pssst: Implants can stop this, and even reverse it.)

Lesson 5

The blame game: the person you see in the mirror.

Maybe as a child, nobody took you to the dentist.

Maybe as an adult, you were raising a family and were too focused on their teeth to worry about your own.

Some people just didn't get around to seeing their dentists or just didn't have time to worry about their oral health.

Some had to make hard choices—between providing for loved ones and going to the dentist.

The result?

A lot of people are missing a lot of teeth, and a lot of them blame themselves.

Missing teeth today are nearly guaranteed to mean more missing teeth tomorrow.

It's time to stop blaming.

Start your new life with a big, healthy smile.

Lesson 6

Take care of your mouth, and it will take care of you.

There's a strong connection between a healthy mouth and good health in general.

All the dieting and exercising in the world are not going to overcome an unhealthy mouth.

A healthy body can't save your mouth.

But, with the advent of dental implants, it's never too late to have that healthy mouth, either.

Because doing something about your teeth is a lot like going to the gym.

It's the same as doing something for your legs, core, or arms.

Or your heart.

Except it's mouth maintenance.

Lesson 7

Congratulations.

You've been putting off tooth replacement.

In the olden days, if you lost a single tooth, you could get fitted for a bridge, which often requires grinding down the two adjoining teeth next to the missing or failing tooth.

This often means you're sacrificing two good teeth in order to replace a bad one.

If you've lost more than one adjacent tooth, you could choose partial dentures.

Back then, those were really your only options.

And not good options, because they don't solve the basic problem: Without the presence of a tooth and its root, the bone in between the remaining teeth will deteriorate, eventually destroying the bridge or requiring larger and larger partial dentures as adjacent teeth weaken and fall out.

Fortunately, now dental implants—single or multiple—fill both primary functions of natural teeth. They support replacement teeth, and they stimulate the underlying bone and keep it healthy.

Be glad you waited.

Lesson 8

The things you'll do for your terrible teeth.

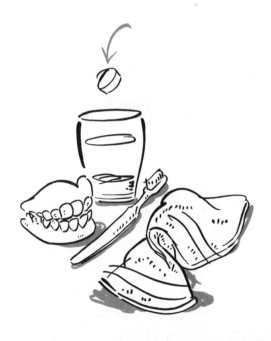

Every day, people go through extraordinary effort and cost to deal with missing teeth, failing teeth, sore gums, dentures, and other dental problems that often could be corrected permanently and quickly.

They bring brushes, picks, mouthwashes, and more to work.

They carry denture adhesive in their pockets and pocketbooks.

They give up their favorite foods.

They chew on one side of their mouths.

They eat only with certain people.

They hide a bunch of accessories in their pocket when they go to a restaurant.

They think no one notices all sorts of picks and flosses.

They hide.

They cope.

Or try to.

But they know the truth.

Even with the best routines, people jump through hoops, give up the foods they love the most, and risk constant embarrassment.

Lesson 9

It doesn't have to get worse.

But it probably will.

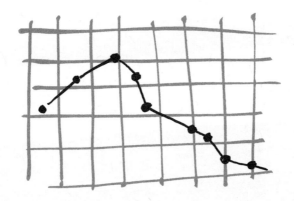

Life with missing teeth or with dentures and "workarounds" is bad enough.

But that's not the whole story.

It's likely to get worse.

There are very few dental problems that "stay the same" over time. (In fact, what is now a "problem" likely used to be an "annoyance.")

There are usually more lost teeth. There is usually more pain. There is usually more movement.

There is usually more coping.

If you've had dentures for several years, your dentures probably don't fit like they did that first year, because you don't have the same jawbone structure to support them.

Any problem that you have now likely means you will be laughing and smiling a lot less later.

And you'll cover up a lot more.

Lesson 10

What are dental implants?

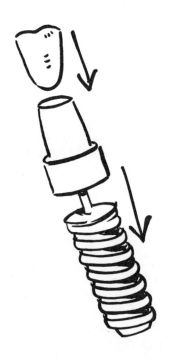

Dental implants are permanent teeth.

They typically have three parts.

1. The implant: A titanium screw that serves as a root for your new teeth. This is inserted permanently into the jawbone and is usually made of high-grade metal such as titanium. The advantages of medical-grade titanium (like that used in knee and hip implants) are that it doesn't corrode and it has properties that help it fuse permanently with human bones. Osseointegration it's called.

   And, more importantly, the implant stimulates the bones and nerves that keep your jaws healthy.

2. The abutment: A permanent (but removable by your doctor) connector that supports a replacement crown (or bridge) that holds a tooth or a set of teeth.

3. The crown: The part of the tooth that you can see. It's usually made of porcelain for good looks. And it's strong, so you can bite into an apple or an ear of corn.

   And so that you can chew anything—even a juicy barbecued steak.

Lesson 11

Who needs dental implants most?

Dental implants are for people missing one, several, or all of their teeth—no matter how they were lost.

Except, that is, for young people under 16 years old, because their jaws are still growing. (Sorry, but many good things are worth waiting for.)

The miracle is that people who have lost or are missing teeth can have them replaced— or restored—with dental implants.

This is true even for people who have lost most of their teeth or who need to have many unhealthy teeth removed.

It's even true for people who never had great teeth in the first place.

And it's especially true for people who are in constant pain, or who suffer constant embarrassment from dentures or dental appliances.

There is now hope for all these people: permanent replacement teeth that are your teeth.

That's really good news!

Lesson 12

For permanent dental implants, see the specialists.

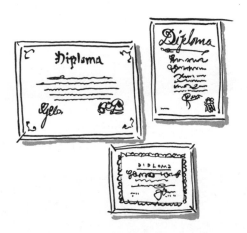

Smiling Lessons

When you're serious about dental implants, it's wise to see people who are just as serious about them: oral surgeons and prosthodontists.

Your oral surgeon is the surgery specialist. They've gone beyond the four-year dental school program required for dentistry to complete at least four more years of a surgical hospital residency. They specialize in treating injuries and diseases of the mouth, jaw, teeth, neck, and gums.

Your prosthodontist is a specialist in the restoration and replacement of teeth, usually with dentures and implants, although also with partial bridges and other appliances.

He or she has gone beyond the four-year dental school program to complete at least three years of additional training in the replacement of missing teeth and the restoration of natural teeth.

So the prosthodontist is really the designer and architect of new teeth. The oral surgeon is like the carpenter.

You and your team work together to design your implants.

You choose the size, color, shape, and imperfections of your new teeth.

They'll look perfect because they're just a bit imperfect. Super-perfect teeth look fake, while imperfect teeth look real.

Lesson 13

The CAT's got your teeth.

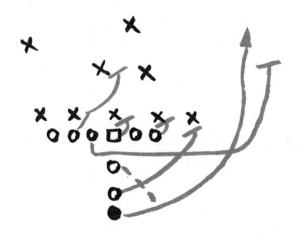

Your doctors will want a 3D CAT (computer-aided tomography) scan made of your mouth and jaws.

That's because in order to plan the work you need, they must know exactly how your bones are structured and how your jaws come together.

Your 3D CAT scan is a sophisticated, computerized, three-dimensional and cross-sectional X-ray of exactly what is going on with your teeth, gums, and bones—along with how they relate to each other.

Your doctors use the scan to decide on the best course of treatment and to design your implants, abutments, and new teeth.

They especially want to make sure that when your implants are anchored, they stay that way.

Lesson 14

Bone grafting.

Fortunately, you probably won't need it.

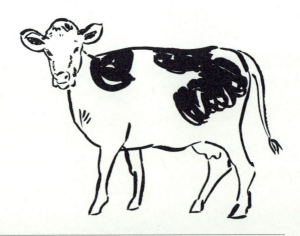

In the early days of implants, if your jawbones were thin or deteriorated (as a result of missing teeth or dentures), bone grafting was necessary. This entailed slicing off a thin chunk of your hipbone or knee bone or part of your jaw and adding it to your upper or lower jaw, or both.

Sometimes it required bone from a donor.

Or from a cow.

Grafting is major surgery, especially when getting multiple implants.

It is done to enlarge and strengthen the bone structure of the jaws.

Grafting was usually done four to eight months before the implant procedure to allow the graft to heal before the implant process disturbs it.

It takes a long time.

And, if replacing all the teeth in a jaw, you'd have to wear dentures for months while it healed.

And walk on crutches while your hips or knees healed.

Sound fun?

Well, don't worry. New advances in implant dentistry make this rarely necessary.

Lesson 15

Early implants were a breakthrough, but they took forever to heal.

When implants arrived on the dental scene more than two decades ago, the good news was that they gave new hope to a lot of people who had given up a lot of foods—and a lot of other things they loved.

The bad news was they required drilling up to two dozen holes in your upper and lower jaws.

Every one of which had to heal.

Because if you put chewing pressure on bones that haven't had time to heal from all these many holes, you would not be in a good place.

So you needed to wait.

And during the healing, usually between six months and a year, you had to wear dentures.

Which has been compared to chewing food with a mouthful of big pink rubber erasers glued into your mouth.

Progress, but with a price.

Lesson 16

You can get a whole new set of teeth in just one day.

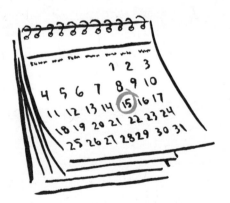

For a full set of new teeth, the earliest implant designs required dozens of implants to be placed into dozens of holes drilled into the jaw, which, of course, required months of recovery time.

Dentures required.

Often, grafting required.

Not anymore.

Using modern techniques, it's likely that you won't need to endure the annoyance, suffering, and embarrassment of wearing dentures while your gums and jaws heal.

These new techniques require as few as four implants to support a whole new set of teeth, which means something amazing:

In most cases, you can have your old, painful teeth removed and your new implants installed the very same day.

You'll wake up to a whole new world, a new set of teeth, and in many cases, you'll be able to chew with them the very first day.

Lesson 17

Yes, you read that right: You can chew the very first day.

One of the most amazing things about the latest implants is that they can go to work for you immediately—many kinds can be used to chew real food the same day they're implanted.

This means you get them in the afternoon and can eat with them that same night.

With minimal recovery time.

You can eat your favorite foods.

You can kiss your favorite person.

No grafting.

No crutches.

No waiting.

And before long, you'll hear yourself saying something astonishing:

"I'd like a second ear of corn, please."

Lesson 18

All gain.
No pain?

The first big reason you can start using modern implants for eating almost immediately comes from breakthroughs in design, materials, and procedures.

You now get stronger teeth, faster, with a minimum number of implant anchors, or holes, drilled in your jaws.

Less surgery usually results in less pain and a quicker procedure.

And you can be blissfully sedated—or sleeping—for the entire encounter.

The second reason is that the level of pain from modern implant techniques is usually less than with earlier methods of treatment.

In fact, given that it's a significant procedure, people expect some discomfort, but many use over-the-counter remedies rather than prescription pain medication.

And only for a couple of days.

Lesson 19

Double trouble.

When you're missing a single tooth, the old way of repairing it was to carve up the adjacent teeth and fashion a bridge between the two, which held the third tooth.

This compromises those two adjacent teeth and does nothing to replace the missing root.

When you lose a tooth, you really need a single implant with a crown—which looks exactly like a tooth. This implant replaces the lost tooth and its root, and prevents the inevitable, debilitating bone deterioration that follows a tooth loss.

When you're missing multiple teeth, implant-supported bridges can replace them. Dental implants can replace both the teeth and the roots—strengthening the jawbones—and can stop or reverse bone degeneration.

When you're missing many or all of your teeth, or need to have several removed, an implant-supported full arch can replace them.

Lesson 20

Always ask for imperfect implants.

You can get perfect crowns, and maybe implants, from your dentist.

That's the first problem.

Perfect teeth look phony. Natural teeth aren't perfect. So it takes the trained eye, and hand, of someone who creates new teeth every day to make them look just a little bit perfectly imperfect.

The second problem is you might want someone who's an expert in facial surgery—an oral surgeon—to do your oral surgery and to make sure that your gums and bone will heal properly.

The third problem is that you really want someone who does implant surgery all day every day to do yours, because you want to have your new teeth for the rest of your life, and you want them done right.

You want someone who'll stand behind you, so your teeth won't cost you any more time or trouble.

But how do you find the right people?

Lesson 21

The referral runaround.

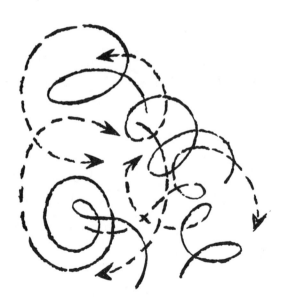

You could see your dentist, who could refer you to an oral surgeon for an oral examination.

Then you'd have to make an appointment, and go.

The oral surgeon would then give you a referral to a 3D CAT scan lab to get a 3D picture of the condition of your jaws and teeth.

Then you'd have to make an appointment, and go.

The CAT scan lab would then send the scan to the oral surgeon to have a look.

The oral surgeon would then refer you to a prosthodontist to make the prosthesis.

Then you'd have to make an appointment, and go.

The prosthodontist would then send you back to the oral surgeon to have the implants seated.

Then you'd have to make an appointment, and go.

Which means that someone has to make all those appointments, and keep them.

That would be you.

Lesson 22

The secret costs of implants.

All those offices and all those appointments on all those days with all those people can require a lot of your time and money.

Typically this runaround not only takes months, but it can cost a lot.

Hidden in those charges are the costs of maintaining separate offices, different staffs, computer and billing systems, and other costs associated with running a professional office.

Or four.

You'll probably have to pay out of pocket, because most healthcare and dental insurance coverage does not cover dental implants.

And every step of the way, the responsibility is yours.

Lesson 23

The decreasing cost of increasing self-esteem.

The good news is that just a few years ago, a full dental replacement with implants could easily have cost $100,000.

But materials, procedures, and costs have fallen dramatically.

So today, your costs are likely to be far lower.

The bad news is that if you wait, your situation, your teeth, and your health are likely to deteriorate.

Your costs are likely to increase.

And what could be a relatively minor procedure now could turn into major surgery later.

Lesson 24

One roof is better (and cheaper) than four.

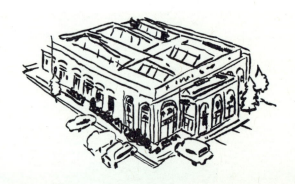

Today, many implant teams work together in the same place with the same goals and tools.

Everything and everyone you need to get your implants are there in one office—all under one roof.

Working together.

This can save you a lot of time, trouble, and money.

But you have to make sure about a few things.

Do they have the most modern 3D CAT scan equipment so they can measure your mouth accurately?

Do they have an on-site lab so they can make and fit your implants quickly?

Do they have both a prosthodontist and an oral surgeon working as a team on-site?

Do they treat your entire case, no matter how big or small, as a single patient file with one person to pay and one person to call with questions?

Lesson 25

Forever is no place for amateurs.

If you're really lucky, or really smart, you won't stop until you find people who've done hundreds, perhaps thousands, of modern implant procedures just like the one you want.

People who work as a team and use the latest tools and techniques, so they can save you a lot of time, aggravation, pain—and, of course, money.

People who can assure that when you go through the process of choosing permanent implants that it's a happy, successful experience.

One that lasts for the rest of your life.

People who make sure that you get a treatment coordinator who explains and helps you through every step of the process.

People who give you a single cost estimate, in writing, at the beginning.

People who stand behind their work, so, in the unlikely event that there's ever an issue they'll be there to handle it.

Lesson 26

Change your mind about your mouth.

With your new implants, you won't see results after a few weeks or months like with a weight-loss or workout program.

You'll see them in seconds—when you wake up and your prosthodontist hands you the mirror.

Implants offer immediate, significant change for almost every element of your life, and the procedure often takes just one day.

You'll feel better about yourself.

You'll feel better about going out in public.

You'll feel better with intimacy in private.

You'll feel better at restaurants, at barbecues, and at business lunches.

But the most important time when you'll feel better is every time you look at your smiling face in the mirror.

Lesson 27

Do you really get to live happily ever after?

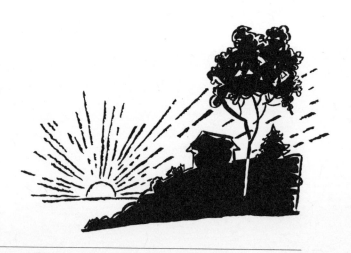

Yes.

Your natural teeth require daily care, brushing, flossing, and regular dental visits.

The same is true of your implants. They require the same care as the original equipment you were born with to keep them clean and to make sure they're good for the rest of your life.

After you've got your implants, your oral surgeon and prosthodontist will work with you to make sure that your implants, teeth, and gums are maintained in good, healthy condition.

So they last as long as you do.

The questions to ask before choosing someone to bring back your smile.

- For me, are there options other than dental implants?
- Why am I a good candidate for dental implants?
- How many appointments will it take for me to get my implants?
- How long have you been placing implants?
- How many implants have you actually placed?
- Do you have reference patients I can hear from?
- What type of sedation will you use?
- Will I need temporary dentures, and if so, for how long?
- Will I need grafting, and if so, from where?
- What are the risks involved?
- How much pain and discomfort can I expect?
- What happens if an implant fails or I need repairs?
- How will you help me with follow-up care?
- What will be the final cost of my treatment, and can I have that in writing?
- Do you have payment plans to help me if I need them?
- Will there be any maintenance required once I have my dental implants?